Foley Catheter Care Plan

A Guide to Indwelling Catheter Care and Reducing Bladder Problems

Written By: Phyllis Irene Hall

Foley Catheter Care Plan Copyright © 2016 by Phyllis Irene Hall - All rights reserved.

No part of this publication may be reproduced, distributed, or transmitted in any form or by any means, including photocopying, recording, or other electronic or mechanical methods, without the prior written permission, except in the case of brief quotations embodied in critical articles or reviews.

Disclaimer

Although the author and publisher have made every effort to ensure that the information in this book was correct at press time, the author and publisher do not assume and hereby disclaim any liability to any party for any loss, damage, or disruption caused by errors or omissions, whether such errors or omissions result from negligence, accident, or any other cause.

The information herein is offered for informational purposes solely, and is universal as so. The presentation of the information is without contract or any type of guarantee assurance.

The trademarks that are used are without any consent, and the publication of the trademark is without permission or backing by the trademark owner. All trademarks and brands within this book are for clarifying purposes only and are owned by the owners themselves, not affiliated with this document.

This book is not intended as a substitute for the medical advice of physicians. The reader should regularly consult a physician in matters relating to his/her health and particularly with respect to any symptoms that may require diagnosis or medical attention.

TABLE OF CONTENTS

Introduction 1

Chapter 1 3
    Urinary catheter: An Overview 3
    Urinary catheter 3

Chapter 2 6
    Types of Catheter 6
    Catheter sizes 6
    Material used in catheters 7
    Foley catheters 8
    Catheter types 10
    Intermittent catheterization 10
    Safety concerns 11
    Drawback of intermittent catheterization 12
    Indwelling catheter 14
    Problems with Foley catheter 15
    Condom catheters or External catheters 16
    Choosing the right external catheter 16
    Suprapubic and urethral catheters 19

Chapter 3 20
    Drain bags 20
    Choosing drainage bag 20
    Leg bags 21
    Tips on using leg bags 21

Bag holders 22

Foley Catheter Legband Holder 22

StatLock Foley Catheter Holder 23

Chapter 4 24

Care of indwelling catheter 24

Removing or attaching leg bag 24

Emptying bag 25

Cleaning leg bag 26

Changing the leg bag 26

Obtaining urine samples 27

Leakage of urine 29

Chapter 5 32

Types of problems associated with catheter use 32

Urinary tract infection symptoms 32

Additional complications 34

Prevention of UTI due to catheter use 35

Use of prophylactic antibiotics 35

Chapter 6 36

When to call your doctor 36

When to get emergency medical aid 36

Portable urinal kits for men and women 37

Having sexual intercourse, while using an indwelling catheter 37

Conclusion 39

Introduction

One of the common problems related to the urinary system include bladder dysfunction, which leads to retention of urine or incontinence. The dysfunction in the bladder results in retention of urine where the bladder is unable to empty urine properly. Urinary incontinence (UI) is the unwanted or involuntary urine leakage.

You have many devices and products, which serve as good treatment options for managing the bladder dysfunction. These devices and products are of immense use to women and men of all age groups. Further, these allow disabled and older individuals to take care of themselves independently. The urinary catheter is one such device that is of significant use in individuals suffering from dysfunction of urinary bladder. Catheter is a thin flexible tube that is passed into the bladder. Urinary catheterization is essentially a medical treatment that involves introducing a catheter into the bladder for draining urine.

Catheterization in general refers to introduction of a catheter into any body cavity for removing or injecting fluid. Urinary catheterization is done to reduce risk of damage to kidneys and infection by ensuring the complete emptying of bladder regularly. Thus, it is used in people diagnosed with bladder obstruction or urinary retention.

Home health care patients use these urinary catheters for various reasons. The use of urinary catheterization is said to date as far back as 300 AD or more. However, the precursor of the present catheter we use now was first used in 1779 and made of gum elastic. Later the catheter was made of latex in 1800s.

The first ever, indwelling catheter was developed by Jean Francois Reybard in 1853. He used an inflated type of balloon to secure the catheter in the bladder. This model was later redesigned by Fredrick Foley in 1932 and today this is the most commonly used device in urinary dysfunction. You have various other types that have evolved since then and with them the management and care of the catheter too has improved. For best patient outcomes, and to avoid complications, proper care of the catheter is very important. This ebook provides a guide on the different types, sizes and materials of catheter, the options present and the associated complications and other related factors. It also provides the best approaches for assessing and managing the catheters in individuals with urinary dysfunction.

Chapter 1

Urinary catheter: An Overview

In the United States alone approximately four million people undergo urinary catheterization in a year and most of these procedures involve use of indwelling catheters. The catheters are placed during hospitalization, especially in residents belonging to long-term health care facilities or home care services.

Urinary catheter

Urinary catheter is a hollow flexible tube used for collecting urine from bladder. It is available in different types and sizes. The materials used for the catheter include latex, rubber or silicone. The tube is connected to the drainage bag, which holds the urine collected. The catheters are used only when the person is unable to empty her or his bladder. If emptying of bladder is disrupted, retention of urine occurs, leading to increased pressure in the kidneys. This may end in kidney failure, which can have fatal consequences as permanent damage to the kidneys may occur.

In general, catheters are used only for a short span, until the person involved is able to urinate independently. However, in case of persons with permanent injury, severe illnesses or elderly people the catheters may have to be used for a longer period.

Use of urinary catheter

Urinary catheters are recommended by a health care professional in case of the following conditions

- Urinary incontinence- This is a condition where there is leakage of urine or inability of the person to control when urinating

- Urinary retention- This condition involves inability to empty bladder
- Surgery in the genitals or prostate
- Spinal cord injury, dementia and multiple sclerosis

Inability to urinate independently may be due to many reasons including,

- Blocked urine flow due to presence of blood clots, bladder stones or narrowing of urethra, which is the narrow tube that links the bladder to the outer part of the body.
- Hysterectomy, repair of hip fracture and surgery on prostate gland
- Injury caused to the nerves present in the bladder
- Medications that affect the muscles of the bladder, leading to impaired squeezing which causes retention of urine.

Catheter usage

A catheter can be used for short term or for long-term basis too.

Short-term catheter use and short-term indications include

If bladder emptying is blocked due to some obstruction like bladder stone

To drain bladder before or after a surgical procedure like prostatectomy or hysterectomy

To monitor output of urine in persons who are recovering from a surgery or are unconscious

To drain bladder before a caesarean birth in women

To clear blood clots or debris in the bladder after injury to it

Long-term indications

For treatment of incontinence, which involves inability to control passing urine or leaking urine, when failure of other treatment procedures occur

Urinary retention where emptying of bladder is not possible

Obstruction in urinary tract due to swollen prostate or bladder stone, when other treatment modalities like medications or surgery cannot be done, to remove obstruction immediately

Nerve damage to bladder, which results in inability to empty bladder also, needs long term catheter use. This condition is called as neuropathic bladder

Bed ridden patients who are weak and unable to use a toilet normally

Chapter 2

Types of Catheter

A urinary catheter varies depending on its size, material and on how it is used.

Catheter sizes

Catheters are generally sized in special units termed as French. One French unit corresponds to one third of a millimeter. Catheters are made from sizes starting at 12 FR, which is termed as small to 48 FR (Large) which corresponds to 3-16mm

The catheters also are available in different varieties including catheters with balloons of different sizes and catheters without bladder balloon. Before using the balloon catheter, you need to check how much it can hold by inflating it with water.

Sizes – Indications

Foley catheters are measured in Charrieres, which is also termed FG (French Grade). One Charriere equals one third millimeter in diameter. The appropriate catheter size selection depends on comfort of patient and on how effective it is in draining the bladder. For instance, a catheter of 12 Ch can drain about 100 liters in a span of 24 hours.

While selecting catheters, the smallest size that enables effective drainage should be used. Large sized catheters are liable to cause mucosal irritation and trauma. However, in case of postoperative bleeding or infection, a larger gauge reduces any risk due to obstruction.

Here is an approximate usage guide on the size of catheter to be used in specific conditions

In females during initial catheterization, clear urine without any presence of debris, grit or hematuria a catheter size of 10 to 12 Ch or 3.3 millimeter should be used.

- For males during initial catheterization, clear urine without any debris, hematuria or grit, a catheter size of 12 to 14 Ch or 4 mm is indicated

- In males during initial catheterization, where the urine is clear or a bit cloudy with mild grit or hematuria with little or no minor blood clots, a size of 16 Ch or 5.3 mm is used

- In males during initial catheterization the presence of moderate or heavy debris, grit or hematuria with clots of moderate size a catheter of 18 Ch or 6 millimeter is used

- Urine that is very cloudy with heavy debris, grit or hematuria with heavy or moderate blood clots, which is usual after prostatic or bladder surgery a catheter size of 20 Ch or 6.7 millimeter, is used.

In case of severe hematuria with large sized blood clots after prostatic or bladder surgery a larger sized catheter of Ch 22 or 7.3 mm should be used

It is recommended to seek guidance from urological health care professionals before using the Charriere sizes. Small sized catheters are generally used in children. While replacing a catheter its size should be noted. While prescribing catheters, the length differs in males and females.

Material used in catheters

Different polymers have been used in the manufacture of catheters. These include silicone rubber, nylon, nitinol, PETE (polyethylene terephthalate), Thermoplastic elastomers and polyurethane. Of these materials, silicone is the commonly used material, as it is inert and does not react with body fluids or any other medical fluids with which it comes in contact. However, at the same time this polymer is mechanically weak resulting in occurrence of serious fractures. The silicone used in Foley catheters has fractured in some cases resulting in surgery being performed to remove the fractured tip present in the bladder.

Easy Insertion

Catheters used in bladder problems now are made of polyurethane, especially the intermittent type of catheter. This is available in different sizes and lengths for women, men and children. The advanced catheter forms contain thin hydrophilic coating on their surface. This coating swells when the catheter is immersed in water forming a smooth and slipper film making it easier to insert and are safer. There are catheters packed in a solution of sterile saline for better and safe insertion.

Foley catheters

Originally, latex rubber was used in Foley catheters. However, this material is obsolete now. While the latex is inexpensive and flexible to use, it has the big drawback of being susceptible to infection and certain hypersensitivity reactions.

While silicone latex is identical to the latex rubber, the silicone added over the latex prevents any endothelial irritation, lacerations or stricture development present in latex. For patients who are exhibit allergic reactions to latex, the superficial silicone layers serves as a protection. However, in some cases the layer of silicone is damaged after some time with the latex material underneath making contact with urothelium. Thus, if the silicone catheters are used, they should be done only for a period of one or two weeks, and should be replaced or removed after that particular span. Hydrogel is also used over latex in some cases instead of silicone.

Only silicone

Foley catheters made of just silicone where all the latex underneath is replaced with silicone is also in use now. However, it is nearly 5 to 10 times more expensive when compared to latex silicone. But due to rise in its popularity the prices have come down now. The main advantage of this material is its long durability for a span of six to eight weeks, while there are manufactures who claim that it can be used for nearly three months. The rigidity of the material is another key benefit.

Since the balloon has the tendency to empty fast due to water loss caused by the semi membranous nature of the balloon wall, it will have to be refilled periodically. And due to the longer life, the tip of the catheter may be covered by encrustations, which constrict the orifice largely or increase the catheter's diameter. This leads to bleeding and pain on removal. Therefore, the catheter should not be left for longer than the time span recommended.

Antimicrobial coating

Catheters have also been constructed with a coating of materials that have antimicrobial properties. This is intended to prevent the biofilm as well as encrustation problems. Silver alloys have been used for this purpose and termed as silver catheters and there are also antibiotic or electrified catheters made in this way. While silver oxide was initially used, later silver alloys with more antimicrobial efficiency were developed.

Catheter choice

The choice of the type of catheter used depends on the purpose it is indicated for. Here are some instances

- In case of preoperative catheterization for simple procedures or in patients who are hospitalized and need catheterization for short span only, silver catheter is the preferred choice. This is because of the antimicrobial property of silver, which helps in avoiding the risk of UTI (Urinary Tract Infection) due to the catheter. But since it is expensive, it is a bit of a drawback.

- Nelaton catheter, which is a straight modeled catheter made from PVC is used in case of simple and short span use like bladder emptying or taking urinary specimen for catheterization. This catheter has a big lumen for rapid flow of urine and does not have any retention facility.

- In case of catheter placement, indwelling Foley catheter is the best choice. A Foley catheter made of silicone is the used as it is more durable than the latex silicone material. Hence, for long-term use, silicone is the material of choice.

- Triple lumen type of catheters is used commonly for irrigation of the bladder continuously, which is needed after surgery in the bladder or prostate.

Catheter tips are available in different forms. The straight tipped model is the standard form used frequently. There are curved tip designs like the Coude or Tiemann type, which are used for easy passage into prostate. This may however run the risk of causing false passages and cause damage. Another model is the whistle tip catheter, which has a lateral opening and one above the balloon to drain the blood clots and debris.

Catheter types

The indication will influence the choice of catheter:

Catheter choice is based on how they are used and is divided into three main categories namely

1. Indwelling catheters - This has two subtypes namely urethral and suprapubic
2. Intermittent catheters
3. Condom or external catheter

Intermittent catheterization

When the catheter tube is passed into and out of bladder intermittently, it is termed as intermittent catheterization. This is done in case of persons who find it difficult to empty their bladder completely. These individuals are taught to use the intermittent catheters.

Catheters generally come with drainage bag for collecting the urine. In case of bedridden patients, the bag is draped over the bedside and in patients who are ambulatory, the bag is attached to the leg with the help of elastic bands. The bag is emptied when needed into a toilet.

In case of intermittent catheterization, the catheter is to be inserted and removes several times in a day. This eliminates using the draining catheter continuously. Although using this type of catheter may seem daunting initially, the process is very simple once you learn it. Most individuals get used to catheterizing themselves and even children seven or eight years of age can be given training to handle the procedure by themselves. If an individual is unable to do it on his own, a caregiver or parent can help.

Effective procedure

This is an effective choice in case an individual is unable to empty bladder on his own. Since leaving urine in the bladder for long periods can lead to distention and urinary tract infection, the procedure helps to prevent such issues. This may also improve urinary incontinence in some cases. Since the catheter is removed after emptying the bladder, a person can take up an active lifestyle than when compared to the indwelling models.

Safety concerns

The long term or indwelling catheters have many side effects due to the long span including blockage, infection, leaking and bladder spasms. The side effects are markedly reduced in intermittent catheterization. When you learn the procedure, it is easy and safe and you need not worry about hurting yourself. The improved lifestyle is another big advantage in this type of catheterization.

Indication

Intermittent catheterization is recommended for patients who are suffering from incontinence, urinary retention and severe bladder conditions, which can cause damage to kidneys. Patients with injury to spinal cord, spina bifida and certain neurological conditions are also prescribed this form of catheterization. This form is also used temporarily for prostate and genital surgery and after abdominal hysterectomy procedure.

Any scar tissue, inflammation, pelvic injury or disease can cause urethra to narrow resulting in difficulty of urine passage. Neurogenic causes including disease of (CNS) central nervous system or in the peripheral nerves, which control the urination reflex, are also indicated. In case of vesico-ureteral reflux wherein the urine flow is reversed and flows from bladder to kidneys or ureters, the intermittent catheterization is recommended.

Mode of action

The sterilized tube or catheter is inserted into urethra, which connects the genitals to bladder. The tube should then be gently guided into bladder, which causes urine to flow via the tube into the bag. When the urine flow stops, you should move it slightly to check for any residual urine. Once bladder is emptied, it can be removed.

Drawback of intermittent catheterization

Based on the reason for using this form of catheterization, the urine may have to be measured and recorded. The drainage bag should be maintained properly and the supplies should be kept track of closely to ensure you have all you need, while doing the procedure. The learning also takes some time, as inserting the catheter past sphincter muscles is difficult. Women too find it hard to insert the catheter. In rare cases, the catheter may rupture the urethral wall causing bleeding, which should be attended immediately.

Types

The use and frequency is advised by the concerned doctor. Catheters used for intermittent catheterization comes in different sizes and types. There are sterile and reusable catheters.

Additional supplies including sanitizers and lubricants are also available for easy use of the catheters.

The common types include Coude intermittent catheter and straight Intermittent catheters

Coude - These are flexible catheters, which possess an elbow or bend curvature. This is to help in easy insertion of the catheter into the urethra in males. These are also indicated in women who have narrowed urethra or block in the urethra. The coude tip is generally used in cases where the straight catheters are not suitable.

Straight – This intermittent catheter is flexible with a rounded and straight tip and sometimes has an opening on the lateral part of the tube

Robinson catheter- This is a catheter with a straight tip. It has about two holes to six holes for increased urine drainage. This is indicated in both female and male patients and indicated especially in patients with obstructed urethral opening due to blood clots

Sizes

The sizes to be used should always be consulted with the physician giving primary care.

Diameter of catheter

This should be large to allow urine to flow freely, but at the same time small to prevent damage to urethra. French catheter scale is used to assess the diameter size, which starts from 3F to 34 F (1 mmm to 11.3 mm) while the common sizes used are in between 10F and 28 F (3.3mm- 9.3mm)

Length of catheter

This varies for males and females. Women need shorter catheter of about 6 inches, while men need 12 inches to 16 inches in length, due to the long urethra present.

Indwelling catheter

This is used in case of continuous bladder drainage conditions. The catheter is stabilized in the bladder with the help of a balloon. The balloon is inflated after inserting to be retained in the bladder. When it is needs to be taken out, the balloon should be deflated.

The indwelling catheters are of two types namely, long-term, which are used for conditions that need catheterization for over 30 days, and short term where the catheter is placed for a term of less than 30 days. The indwelling catheter collects the urine in a draining bag attached to it. There are also newer catheter types, which are fitted with valves that help in draining the urine out easily.

Indwelling catheter is inserted in the bladder by two methods:

Urethral catheterization: This is the most common method used for draining urine. The catheter passes via the urethral tube, which connects the bladder to the exterior and it the normal route for passage of urine.

Suprapubic catheterization: This is an alternative method where a minor surgery is performed to create an artificial track to the bladder via the lower part of abdomen. For long-term catheterization, this is the most preferred method.

Foley catheter

Foley catheter is an indwelling catheter that helps in creating a safe passage for draining and collecting urine. The pliable material it is made of helps it to indwell into the bladder via urethra. The catheter has two channels present separately in the tube allowing a safe extraction and good stability when inserted. One of the channels is stabilized in the bladder with the help of a balloon. The second channel lets passage of urine and its collection in the drainage bag present on the bedside or in a leg bag strapped to the leg of the person.

Foley catheters are generally made of latex or silicone. The catheters should be used as per instructions of the physician in charge of the primary care of the patient.

Placement of Foley Catheter

The deflated balloon end of the catheter is inserted into urethra and moved gently and slowly. The patient needs to take slow and deep breaths and push as when trying to urinate, while insertion is done.

Lubricant jelly is applied on the Foley catheter to facilitate smooth entry. Once urine flows from the Foley catheter the balloon is filled to hold the catheter in a stable position and prevent it from coming out. The open catheter end is attached to a drainage bag.

Problems with Foley catheter

Some of the difficulties that some patients may experience with the catheter include

- Urine does not drain into the bag: You need to straighten out any kinks present in the catheter tubing. The strap should be checked on whether it is blocking the tube. Ensure that you are not lying or sitting on the tube. The urine bag should be present below waist level.

- Urine leaks from tubing, drainage bag or around the Foley catheter: Check for accidental opening of closed drainage part of the tubing. The catheter and its ends should be cleaned with alcohol pad and reconnected.

Risks present

Developing an infection is the highest risk, which can occur when the drainage is opened allowing bacteria to enter the tubing. Improper cleaning of the equipment or not washing hands properly can also cause infection, which can spread on to the bladder and other organs leading to severe consequences.

Condom catheters or External catheters

These are used commonly in elderly men suffering from dementia. Unlike the other catheter types, a tube is not placed inside the penis. A device resembling a condom is placed over the penis. The device is connected to a tube, which connects to the drainage bag. The catheter should be changed daily. The catheter is used just for short spans only.

External or condom catheters are indicated in men to treat conditions like urinary incontinence. The catheter is made of a flexible cover, which slides on the penis similar to a condom. This is a great alternative, when compared to the invasive catheters like indwelling catheters. Other than being a preferred alternative to indwelling catheters, it is also straightforward and easy to use. The catheter needs to be just rolled on the penis and it attaches by an adhesive added to it. There are also external catheters without adhesives like Texas catheters, which use strap of elastic foam or a loop and hook type.

Choosing the right external catheter

While selecting the external catheter that meets your specific needs, you should consider factors like the comfort it offers, the cost, reliability, convenience, sensitivity and security. There are latex and silicone materials used. For those with latex allergy, silicone catheters are preferred and these have integrated adhesive feature. If you do not have latex allergy, the latex catheters can be used.

The latex types do not have an adhesive, and need to be used with a two sided or one-sided strip. These are easy to use and inexpensive but do not give good seal and may trigger allergic reactions.

Silicone catheter is breathable, odor free and does not cause skin irritation. It is also uniformly adhesive. The only drawback is the expensive price.

Indications for external catheters

The condom catheters are mainly prescribed in case of

- Patients with impaired vision, reduced mobility and dementia who have limited access to toilet
- Damaged sphincter caused due to prostatectomy
- Spinal cord injuries leading to reflexive voiding
- Concerns of leaving the patient unsupervised or without assistance, while using the toilet
- Urinary urgency or frequency, which is unmanageable

Condom catheter contraindications

There are very few contraindications present for the use of external catheters and should be considered fully before deciding on its use. The contraindications include

- Sensitivity or allergic reactions to adhesives or latex used in the catheter
- Hypospadias caused by catheter use
- Skin irritation, ulcers, open lesions, paraphimosis, or phimosis in the glans penis

Size determination

To determine the size, the penis circumference should be measured in millimeters and used in the formula- cx7/22 for arriving at the penis diameter. The external catheters are measured by the diameter as 25 mm, 27mm etc.

Instruction for use

The successful use of condom catheter is achieved only when the catheter is applied properly. Ensure that all creams and residual adhesives are removed completely form the penis. The penis should be washed thoroughly using soap and water. The penis should then be dried and the catheter should be applied over the glans penis in its natural position. For those without foreskin this is not an issue.

Moisture barrier creams or other ointments, which disrupt the catheter adhesive, should be avoided. And the constriction of penis and presence of kinks in the catheter should be monitored. Use of adhesive tape on the catheter can lead to penis restriction, catheter inflexibility and damage to penis. Pubic hair should not be shaved to prevent skin irritation.

The duration of use of the condom catheter depends on the type of catheter used and the skin sensitivity of the patient. In general, the duration should be between 12 hours and 72 hours. For removal, the penis is soaked with warm washcloth for 30 seconds. The catheter should be removed daily for skin inspection and cleaning purpose.

Risk factors

Most of the complications in condom catheter use is due to faulty equipment manufacturing and error while using. Proper hygiene along with appropriate use avoids many complications caused by the catheters. The common conditions that occur include bacteriuria, edema, allergic reaction, inflammation in glans penis, allergic reaction and maceration, pruritus, dermatitis and erythema in penis, skin tears and ischemic injury to tissues.

Comparing catheters

Selection of the right catheter depends on the clinical requirements, expected duration of the catheter use, infection risks and patient preference.

External and indwelling catheters

The condom catheters also termed as penile sheath catheters are indicated in men with incontinence and impaired renal function but no urinary retention. These are especially suitable for use during nighttime only. The bacteremia rate is lower and these are more comfortable when compared to indwelling catheters but leakage, risk of skin damage, penile ischemia and urethral diverticula are major drawbacks.

Indwelling and intermittent catheters

In case of patients with neuropathic bladder, intermittent catheterization is preferred as there are no separate systems for collection of urine. The intermittent form is also part of standard care given to patients with injuries in spinal cord. However, it may not be feasible functionally or not acceptable to some patients. The bacteremia levels are reduced in post-operative cases including hip fracture repair and after hysterectomy. The return to normal voiding is also quicker. When used for long-term it may cause bacteremia, but much reduced infection of urinary tract than indwelling catheterization.

In some cases, both types are used in combination to accommodate the individual lifestyles and needs.

Suprapubic and urethral catheters

The suprapubic catheters are more advantageous in terms of convenience and comfort. They can be easily clamped to test the voiding function and offer better sexual function and self-image. However, these catheters have downsides including cellulitis risk, prolapse of urethra and leakage. The insertion also needs higher expertise level.

Chapter 3

Drain bags

A catheter is usually attached to a drainage bag. There are two types of bags: A small sized device called leg bag and a larger one for draining during nighttime. The leg bag is attached with the help of elastic bands. The bag holds around 300 milliliters to 500 milliliters urine. This is mostly worn during daytime as it can be used under a skirt or pant and emptying is easy.

Larger drainage device is for nighttime use mostly and can hold up to 2 liters urine. The device is hanged by the bed or it is placed on the ground.

The drainage bag should always be present at a level below the bladder to prevent urine from flowing back in the bladder. The bag should be drained for every eight hours or when the bag fills up.

For cleaning the bag, it should be removed from its attachment to the catheter. A new drainage bag should be attached to the free catheter, while the old one is cleaned. The bag should be cleaned with a mixture of water and vinegar or chlorine bleach can also be used. The bag should be soaked in the solution for a minimum of 20 minutes. This should then be hanged dry with the outlet valve kept in open position for the bag to dry up easily.

Choosing drainage bag

With a wide variety of drainage systems present, the choice needs to be done based on the needs of the individual and the catheterization method. The urinary drainage bag attached to knee, calf or thigh is the most commonly used system and it has capacities ranging from 350 ml to 750 ml for adults. The body worn drain bags are for daytime use and enable better mobility. Larger capacity bags are for drainage during night. The night bags come with drainage tap to help in emptying and remain for up to seven days. They should be placed using a hanger on the bed or as free standing. Whatever drainage system is used, it is important to maintain a closed system to prevent risk of urinary tract infections.

Leg bags

These are designed for discrete urine storage under clothing and are attached either to a sheath or to catheter. The leg bags are for daytime use. They are strapped to the leg comfortably using support devices or straps.

Tips on using leg bags

If the tubing of the cathcter is sufficiently long so it reaches the ankle, you can empty the bag without removing your trousers. In case you are wearing shorts, thigh bags or a catheter valve can be used. While choosing the leg bag, you should consider the length of the tubing, shape of leg, and strap model and bag position on your leg. The attachment options are varied and are chosen based on where the bag is attached on your leg. For instance, garment holder for leg bag on the calf, and in the thigh, straps, are used. The tubing of the leg bag can be adjusted, according to individual requirements.

While choosing a leg bag, the most important factors to be looked include

- Taps- These should be easy to open without leaking on the fingers when the bag is emptied

- Straps- Should be comfortable

- Proper seal - No leakage should be present in the connectors or bags

Leg bags are also attached to certain types of urinals of hand held type in case more amount of urine storage is needed. If the urine loss is only light and you need leg bag to be connected to just a sheath, there are smaller custom-made bags available.

The leg bags are available with different features, designs and sizes enabling you to choose one that suits your specific needs. Most of the bags are made of good quality and durable vinyl material. These are reusable and leak resistant too. The leg bags are fitted with anti-reflux valve, which ensures that the urine flows into the bag only. Leg bags are now available with comfortable straps for better positioning and easy to drain with valves designed as one-way feature so back flow is prevented.

Bag holders

Catheter bag holders are created to prevent drainage bag from coming into contact with skin. These conceal the bag, support its weight and protect the body by avoiding the bag from contacting with the skin.

There are customized bag holders that offer appropriate solution for concealing and supporting catheter drainage bag. The bag holder is worn on the body and it supports the drainage bag securely. In addition, it provides easy access to drain the bag, if necessary.

There are lower leg bag holders situated near the calf region extending from the knee bottom to over the ankle.

The upper leg bag holder is used in the thigh region. It comes with adjustable closure or as a pull up holder.

Some holders attach around the waist with a vertical pouch that extends over thigh region to support the drainage bag. There are essentially two commonly used bag holders- Foley Catheter Legband Holder and StatLock Foley Catheter Holder.

Foley Catheter Legband Holder

This stabilizes the indwelling catheter and enables greater comfort without limiting movement of the patient. The band is made of 100 percent cotton and comes with a single size that fits all. The holding mechanism is by means of Velcro Locking system, which is easy and quick to engage. The soft and comfortable material allows complete movement range. It wraps around the leg without any need for shaving or use of adhesive. The main advantages include;

- No skin tears produced by the adhesive tape
- Risk of infection and irritation is avoided
- Comes in a single size that fits everyone
- Free of latex, so does not cause any allergic reactions or irritation

StatLock Foley Catheter Holder

This type of Foley Catheter holder is designed to hold the catheter in place without use of leg strap. This holder forms a viable alternative for the strapping type of bag holder with its anchor pad design. The anchor pad is made of latex free material and secures tightly to the skin preventing the bag from slipping. The anchor pads are easier and safe to use, when compared to sutures. The air permeable design of the anchor pads also reduces irritation to the skin.

The holder contains a retainer device, which attaches the anchor pads holding the catheter in place securely. The retainer has transparent gull shaped wings, which hold the catheter. The wings should be lifted and catheter placed inside. Once the catheter is placed, the wings are closed over it. This method is simple and safe and further the holder can turn 360 degrees on its axis. This prevents accidental removal of catheters or pulling on them. This holder fits with most models of latex and silicone catheters.

Advantages of the statlock catheter holder include;

- 360 degree rotation prevents pulling
- Adhesive anchor pad for preventing needle sticks
- Breathable and sterile material made of silicone and is free of latex

Chapter 4

Catheter care

Care of indwelling catheter

Foley catheter passes through urethra into the bladder, where it is held in position by means of a balloon filled with water. To collect urine that passes via the catheter it is attached to a bag on the outside, which is a small sized leg bag or a larger drain bag. The larger bag is used for collection of urine at nighttime. The leg bag is sufficient for daytime use.

Removing or attaching leg bag

The leg bag attached to the thigh, knee or calf allows for, free movement and the bag is hidden under the clothes you wear. This makes you feel comfortable about using the catheter. Removal or attachment of leg bag is as follows

You need supplies including clean leg bag, tape or leg straps, alcohol pads, cotton balls and white vinegar. Water and towel is also needed.

For leg bag removal, here are the steps to be followed

- Wash hands with water and soap for about 15 seconds
- Empty the drainage bag
- A towel is placed under the area where the bag and catheter are connected.
- The rubber tube should be pinched off to prevent urine from leaking out
- The Foley catheter should be disconnected from the drainage bag using twisting motion

- The catheter should not be pulled on while doing this. The used drainage bag should be placed over the towel.

- The leg drain bag's tube tip has a protective coating, which should be removed. The tip is then cleaned with alcohol pad to avoid dirt from getting into the tip.

- The leg bag straps should be fastened to the thigh and catheter secured with tape. The catheter should have some slack to prevent it from exerting pressure on the urethra, bladder and other body parts.

- The straps should not be fastened too tightly on the bag as it may disrupt the circulation. If the strap is dirty, it should be washed using soap and some water.

Emptying bag

Since leg bags are smaller in size, when compared to the regular sized drainage bags they need to be emptied frequently. The leg bag should be emptied minimum twice in a day or when the bag is half-empty.

Place a large metal or plastic container nearby for emptying the urine or it can be emptied directly into the toilet too.

Wash hands using soap and water.

The drain bags open differently based on their type. They may have a draining spout, which you open from the sleeve or a clamp that opens on the side or as an opening that twists. Irrespective of the method used, avoid touching the tip, while you drain the urine into the toilet or container.

After you empty the bag completely, close the drainage bag's clamp and return it to the bottom of the leg bag.

Wash hands using soap and water

If required by your physician, you need to keep a record of the amount of urine in the bag.

Changing the leg bag to the other leg occasionally is a good idea, and this should be done just after you take your bath.

Cleaning leg bag

When you are ready to sleep, the leg bag should be changed with the drainage bag. Rinse the leg bag with three parts of water and one part of vinegar and let it soak for about 20 minutes. Use warm water to rinse it and hang it to dry.

The next day morning, remove the drainage bag and put on your leg bag. Clean the drainage bag similar to what you did for the leg bag.

The leg bag should be cleaned daily and replaced whenever your physician recommends it. This is done generally once in a month.

Changing the leg bag

The leg bag should be changed once in a month or sooner if it appears dirty or smells bad. Here are the steps you need to follow

- Wash hands thoroughly

- Disconnect valve present at the part where the catheter attaches to the bag. Do not pull hard on the valve. The end of the bag or tube should not be allowed to touch any surface or your hands.

- Clean the tube end with alcohol and cotton ball.

- The opening present on the clean bag should also be wiped with alcohol

- Attach the bag with the tube securely

- The bag should be strapped to the leg

- Wash hands thoroughly

Obtaining urine samples

Catheterization is used occasionally to obtain samples of clean urine for detecting any bacterial infections in the urine. The 'clean urine' indicates urine that is not contaminated by the bacteria from your genitals or hands. The sample is collected directly from the bladder with the catheter. To get a sample, you need to use the standard type of drainage bag or the leg bag.

Sample collection

The urine sample collection is done for various reasons including ruling out presence of infection and supervising the hydrated state of the patient.

The sample should be obtained in the same way irrespective of the nature of tests done. The specimens should be collected from the place between the catheter tube and collection bag, and not directly from collection bag. This is because bacteria are prone to develop in the unclean environment of the bag and give unreliable results.

A small sized port is present in the catheter tube, where it nears the collection bag. For obtaining a sample, the port should first be swiped with alcohol swab and urine sample drawn directly from tubing with sterile syringe. Surgical asepsis should be used, while getting the sample, transfer of the sample to sterile cup and covering it with a secure lid and while transporting it. The samples should be labelled with the name, birth date, and time and date the sample had been obtained. The sample should be refrigerated or placed on ice, until they are sent to the laboratory.

Precautions

While using the catheter, liquids should be taken in plenty. A minimum of 8 cups of liquids should be taken, if approved by your primary care physician.

The tubing should not be tugged or pulled. This causes bleeding and damages the area where the balloon filled with water is present in the bladder.

Take care to avoid stepping on tubing, while walking. You can hold the tubing in curled form in your hand and place the drain bag at a level below the bladder while walking. You can also pin or clip the tubing to your clothes.

The catheter tubing should be arranged in such a manner, so it does not loop or twist. While sleeping, you should hang the drain bag by the side of the bed. Sleeping can be done in the position you wish, provided the bedside drain bag is at a level below the bladder. The urine bag should not be placed down on the flooring.

The urine bag functions properly only when it is below the bladder at the level of your waist. If you fail to place it below bladder level, the urine will flow back from urine bag and tubing into bladder leading to infection. While using leg bag avoid going to bed or taking long naps.

While you shower, keep the large drain bag in position and let it hand on a rail nearby. The plug that is present in the area where drainage bag attaches to catheter can also be used. The drainage bag should be covered and set aside while showering. The bag should be reconnected after you shower. Covering the tubing of the drainage bag is important to prevent contamination.

In case you dislodge catheter, it will leak or stop draining. Leakage may be due to other causes like blockage, bladder spasms or dislodgement. You need to call your physician immediately.

The draining tube and catheter should be checked regularly to ensure the tube is not tangled or squeezed.

General care

The area of the catheter that exits from your body should be cleaned regularly with soap and water. The area should also be cleaned after each bowel movement. This will avoid infection risk. In case of suprapubic catheter, the opening in the belly should be cleaned and covered with dry gauze.

Fluids should be had in plenty to avoid infections. You need to ask your primary care provider on the amount of fluids you can take.

Hands should be washed thoroughly after and before you handle the drainage system. The outlet valve should not touch any surface and if it gets dirty, clean the outlet with soap and water.

To reduce infection risk, you need to drink water in sufficient amounts. This will keep the urine slightly yellow hued or clear and aid in preventing infection.

Drainage bag for collecting urine should be fully emptied once in eight hours or whenever it is half-full. A plastic squirt bottle with a mixture of water and bleach or vinegar should be used to clean it.

Leakage of urine

Urine can sometimes leak near the catheter, which is caused due to

- Block in the catheter or kink in the catheter
- Very small catheter
- Spasm in the bladder
- Constipation
- Infection in urinary tract
- Wrong sized balloon

Things to do while having a catheter

When you undertake the necessary precautions, while using the urinary catheter you can be comfortable more and prevent infection to your kidney and bladder. Some of the precautions you take include;

- Avoid removing urinary catheter on your own. If the catheter does not work properly, you should inform your health care provider or doctor immediately. The catheter should be removed only by your physician or nurse in the physician's office. This will ensure that the catheter is removed properly without damaging your bladder or urethra.

- The catheter and skin around it should be kept clean always. Clean the area twice a day and after each bowel movement.

- Wash hands thoroughly both before as well as after you clean the catheter

- The urine drain bag should be present below bladder level at the waist. This helps to prevent urine from flowing into the bladder. If you fail to do this, germs may enter the body causing pain, fever, redness or swelling.

- Cotton underwear should be worn always. This allows proper airflow in the region and keeps the genital area dry.

- Liquids to be taken include milk, water and drinks, which do not contain caffeine. Caffeine should be avoided, as it will cause frequent urination leading to loss of body fluids.

- Sexual intercourse is limited, consult your doctor for recommendations.

- Prevent being constipated, as it will cause you to push hard, which results in urine leak. To prevent constipation, ensure you have fluids in plenty and avoid caffeine. Add fiber to the diet in the form of whole grains, fresh fruits, vegetables and prunes.

- Avoid taking over the counter medications for constipation. Consult with your health care provider or team for medications.

- Avoid eating foods that can cause irritation to the bladder including acidic foods, alcoholic beverages, carbonated drinks, and drinks with caffeine, spicy foods, lemon juice, cranberries, coffee and chocolate. These foods can however be taken after the catheter is removed.

- If you find urine leaking around the region where the catheter exits your body, use gauze to soak it up. If the leakage is more, you should get medical help immediately

- Kegel's exercise should not be done, while the catheter is present

It is normal to pin or clip the catheter tubing to your cloth. Ensure that you do not hurt the tubing with the pin or clip.

Chapter 5

Types of problems associated with catheter use

While catheter use is advised after all other possibilities have been assessed, prolonged or improper use has high infection risk. The risk further increases, if the catheter is placed for a long period as in an indwelling catheter, or if the patient uses the catheter himself. If you are using a catheter on your own, it is important to know the proper use and the appropriate hygiene procedures to be followed, while using the catheter.

Urinary tract infection symptoms

Infection in the urinary tract is the most common risk related to catheter use. The symptoms of infection in the urinary tract include,

- Pain while urinating
- Change in the normal urinating pattern like for instance, urinating much more than the normal amount
- Passing cloudy or foul smelling urine
- High temperature of over 100.4 Fahrenheit or more
- Vomiting

If the above symptoms are present, you need to contact your doctor immediately. Antibiotics are prescribed as a precautionary measure in long-term catheterization to avoid UTIs.

Other issues present

Injury to urethra due to improper insertion of catheter

Narrowing of urethra because of formation of scar tissue due to improper catheter insertion

Bladder injury due to insertion

In long term, may be over several years of catheterization, bladder stones may develop.

Other complications

Complications that arise due to catheter use include

- Sensitivity or allergy to latex
- Septicemia (blood infections)
- Blood in urine (Hematuria)
- Injury to urethra
- Infection in the urinary tract or kidney

The complications that arise are divided into traumatic and infective complications

Traumatic complications

These complications result in injury or damage in the organs due to catheter use. These include formation of false passages, strictures in urethra, perforation of urethra and bleeding.

Infective complications

The infective conditions that result due to use of catheter include, asymptomatic bacteriuria, urethritis, cystitis, epididymitis, epididymo-orchitis, prostatitis, pyelonephritis, vesico-ureteric reflux, septicemia, infection in the abdominal wall, bacteremia and in severe cases septic shock.

UTI risk

Of the various risk factors, risk of urinary tract infection is the greatest in patients using catheter. And this is more during the insertion of catheter. Silicon catheters are preferred over other materials due to their reduced risk. This is because they can be used for longer duration, while other catheters need to be changed frequently causing increased infection risk. However, if intermittent catheters can be used for a particular situation, they should be preferred over indwelling catheters to prevent infection.

Bacteriuria

In an indwelling catheter, the most common infection to occur is bacteriuria, which has an infection percentage of five percent per day, and in one week, it is 50 percent, and in one month, all patients tend to develop the infection. But treatment need not be started, if the patient is asymptomatic except in case of pregnancy, imminent urological surgery and renal transplant surgery that has been done recently.

Long-term bacterial infection may lead to complex microbial colonization and development of poly-microbial infection and biofilm formation. The common pathogen found is Echerichia coli, but you also find staphylococcus saprophyticus, staphylococcus epidermidis and enterococcus species. As long as the catheter remains inside the bladder, the infection will not be cleared by antibiotics, but resistance to infection is increased.

Additional complications

The long-term use of catheter also causes several additional complications including

- Chronic pyelonephritis
- Chronic inflammation in the renal system
- Nephrolithiasis
- Chronic renal failure
- Cystolithiasis
- In rare cases, cancer in bladder

Renal failure

Renal failure has been reported as one of the main causes of fatality in about 68 percent of patients who have had injury in spinal cord. The risk is further increased by urolithiasis. Some of the preventative procedures include renal ultrasound, creatinine clearance and review of urology. For patients who have been catheterized for over 10 years, the increased risk of cancer in bladder is present. Cystoscopy or cytology is recommended annually as preventative procedure.

Prevention of UTI due to catheter use

There are many recommendations by experts on infection control for patients with catheter, which include:

- The long-term use of catheterization should be done only after all other options and considerations are rejected. The need for catheterization should be reviewed regularly.

- The type of catheter used should be selected based on the clinical need of the patient, the span of use, preference of patient and infection risk.

- Bladder washouts should not be used, to prevent infection

- Urethral meatus needs to be kept clean with soap and water

- Aseptic method of catheterization should be used and done only by properly trained professionals

- Antibiotic prophylaxis while catheter changing should be given only in patients with CA-UTI history and those who have endocarditis risk

Use of prophylactic antibiotics

While possible reduction of infection risk has not been recorded in patients who used prophylactic antibiotics, general opinion on use of prophylaxis is that it should be considered only in patients with high risk of endocarditis and CA-UTI. Aminoglycosides or fluoroquinolones (oral) are given in single dose for prophylaxis, and in endocarditis, anti-streptococcal agents are used.

Chapter 6

When to call your doctor

You need to get help from your health care provider, if you find the following signs:

Chills or fever

Bleeding present around or into the catheter

Spasms in bladder that persist

Urine leaking in the region around catheter in large amounts

Skin sores present around the suprapubic-catheter insertion area

Strong smelling urine or cloudy and thick urine

In spite of drinking sufficient amount of fluids, absence of urine or very little amount

The catheter should be replaced at once, if it found to be clogged, infected or painful

In case you see blood in the drainage bag or tubing or find itching or rash where the catheter tube is attached to your skin, you should contact your health care physician.

If the closed drainage opens or pulls apart accidentally, or you see crystal layers inside tubing, you need to seek medical help.

When to get emergency medical aid

Emergency medical care should be availed in case of

- Catheter coming out
- Material like sand present in drainage bag or tubing

- No urine draining into bag even after checking the system properly

- Pain in pelvis, back, hip or lower abdomen region

- Bladder spasms

- You are not able to think clearly or are feeling confused

Portable urinal kits for men and women

Portable urinals for men and women allow a quick, convenient and hygienic choice. These are good choices for patients in non-ambulatory condition. The small sized urinals allow convenience and enhanced independence. They also prevent accidents. The portable urinal kits for women are reusable and are shaped to prevent any urine leaks. The portable urinal kits for men provide discreet and quick bladder relief. There are disposable unisex urinals, which are even better on maintaining hygiene.

The advantages of the portable urinal kits include

Hygienic containment of urine

Provide portable and convenient bladder relief

Available in gender specific as well as unisex disposal units

Having sexual intercourse, while using an indwelling catheter

Most patients are concerned about maintaining their sexual activity, while having indwelling catheter. In case of an indwelling type of catheter, there are two options. The patient can take the catheter out before having intercourse and replace it with a new one after. This is an expensive option. In addition, it is complicated, if they cannot insert it themselves. In some instances, you are taught on removing and replacing catheter safely to have sex easily.

Not replacing it immediately may lead to autonomic dysreflexia or incontinence or infection risk. Another option is to leave the catheter as it is, and tape it to the thigh, so it does not interfere in case of women and in men, a condom can be worn with a large catheter loop left at the end of penis. They can fold catheter tubing along the penis base and cover the penis and tube with condom. The condom is placed to prevent infection of urinary tract due to exposure of catheter at the penis tip. The catheter can be clamped and urine bag emptied, removed, and placed nearby securely to prevent discomfort of its presence.

Conclusion

Urinary catheters offer a good option for monitoring urine output, diagnosing urinary tract infection and most importantly to relieve retention of urine. The convenience of use and universal availability can sometimes lead to prolonged and indiscreet use of catheters.

While condom catheters or external catheters offer a safe alternative, in situations where prolonged catheterization need arises, intermittent catheters help in reducing irritation locally, infection and formation of bladder stone.

The catheters should be handled with proper hygienic methods for safe use. Further selection of small sized catheters and closed drainage devices are preferred to reduce risks present. With the use of catheter being associated with discomfort, trauma in the lower part of urinary tract, calculi formation, spasms in bladder and issues with the balloon in the catheter, minimizing the use of catheter during surgeries is being considered widely.

Due to the high potential of complications related to infection and trauma, using urinary catheters should be limited to only when they are absolutely needed. In men who are able to spontaneously void, the condom catheter drainage should be preferred.

Intermittent self-catheterization is another preferred option as it has fewer risks of infection, bacteriuria, bladder spasm, calculi formation, blocked catheters, leakage and renal failure, which are seen with long duration of catheterization.

For minimizing infection, you need to use systems with closed drainage and catheters of smaller bores. Hygiene is also vital. In case of infection, the condition should be aggressively managed. Catheterization is not needed before and after elective surgeries like pelvic and orthopedic surgeries and in case of diagnostic laparoscopies.

Although urinary catheterization provides a simple yet valuable method that is easily performed by a patient, nurse or physician, the potential risks and complications that it is associated with should be considered before using it. The procedure should be considered only when necessary.

If you do require a urinary catheter for a long term, you need to know in detail about looking after the catheter at home. The various things you require to know include, knowing about getting catheter supplies, reducing infection risk, identifying potential problems and when to **call a doctor for medical advice.**

When you follow instructions carefully, it will be easy to lead a relatively routine normal life. The bag and catheter are easy to conceal under clothes. Almost all day-to-day activities can be done with the catheter including going to work, swimming, having sex and exercise.

While living with a urinary catheter may be a challenging task, you can accomplish it with the right information and help from your health care support group.

Thanks for reading, I hope this book was able to help you manage your catheter care.

Finally, please consider leaving a comment/review for this book on – especially any tips to help other catheter users; it would be greatly appreciated!

P.S. I use an 18fr 30cc Silicone catheter and sediment blocking the line is my biggest problem. My solution is drinking lots of fluids and flushing the line using a piston syringe and saline solution

Subscribe to my newsletter for more Home Healthcare tips: writerpirenehall@aol.com

Printed in Great Britain
by Amazon